Paulo Autran Leite Lima
Milena de J. da Silva
Walderi M. da Silva Júnior

Reducing hospital costs with the use of TENS

Paulo Autran Leite Lima
Milena de J. da Silva
Walderi M. da Silva Júnior

Reducing hospital costs with the use of TENS

Postoperative inguinal hernioplasty

ScienciaScripts

Imprint

Cover image: www.ingimage.com

This book is a translation from the original published under ISBN 978-613-9-62560-4.

Publisher:
Sciencia Scripts
is a trademark of
Dodo Books Indian Ocean Ltd. and OmniScriptum S.R.L publishing group

120 High Road, East Finchley, London, N2 9ED, United Kingdom
Str. Armeneasca 28/1, office 1, Chisinau MD-2012, Republic of Moldova, Europe
Printed at: see last page
ISBN: 978-620-7-73051-3

SUMMARY

Capitulo 1 AN INTRODUCTION TO HOSPITAL COSTS AND PHYSIOTHERAPY RESOURCES

FLAVIO WALLACE DE BRITO PINTO; ANDRÉ SALES BARRETO; PAULO AUTRAN LEITE LIMA

Nowadays, talking about costs is a very worrying subject, given that we are living in a third world country subject to the strong influence of foreign capital. In the Brazilian hospital network, this is alarming, as all the latest equipment and medicines are imported, usually at very high prices related to the exchange rate. Between 2005 and 2016, the pharmaceutical industry was allowed to adjust the prices of its products by up to 77%. It was only in 2016, when inflation was around 10%, that the prices of medicines were adjusted above the average, setting the maximum adjustment allowed to manufacturers at 12.5%.

The increase in hospital costs is due to the rise in the average age of the population, diseases caused by globalization, new technologies for tests and treatments and, consequently, the difficulty of managing these costs in a way that is accessible to the population as they seek quality of life and physical and mental well-being. In view of these expenses, the 2008-2009 Family Budget Survey (POF) pointed to average spending on medicines as the main portion of the population's health expenditure, with a percentage of 77.3% of the Brazilian population.

Cost management needs to be carried out in detail, and in order to reduce expenditure, it is necessary to combine clinical practice with the expenditure that is essential to maintain the quality of the service provided. However, optimizing cost reductions, always seeking to promote the most effective plans and looking for ways to implement technological innovations can help in the thoughtful use of resources, but it is an arduous task, mainly because it is based on large economic models.

Based on studies on the increasing costs, hospitals in both developing and developed countries have proposed the adoption of quality and efficiency programs in the health sector, which are strongly related to the costs of hospital care when compared to the total investment in health.

The current state of the health sector shows the need to deal with advances in research, innovative diagnostic technologies, an increase in the average age of the population, contracts, demands from regulatory bodies, payment negotiations, the constant search for quality, efficiency in treatment and people management.

With the aim of systematizing and comparing the available evidence of alternative technologies in relation to their health outcomes and costs in order to support decision-making regarding the efficient use of available resources, four types of economic evaluation have been developed: cost-minimization, cost-benefit, cost-effectiveness and cost-utility.

Quality programs face obstacles to their introduction, because the laws of the market do not apply well to the hospital sector in view of human needs and non-market priorities. In addition, doctors show great resistance to quality programs, as they are not used to having their work evaluated from the perspective of measuring quality, since they feel supervised and are afraid of losing their autonomy in the clinical management of patients. In addition, the majority of patients are lay people and do not have the ability to judge whether their treatment has been carried out well, making it difficult for them to exercise their consumer choices and reducing prior control of hospital quality.

The limited resources of materials and specialized professionals for the control of healthcare-related infections (HAIs) contribute to outbreaks of fast-growing microbacteria in invasive procedures. This factor, combined with the side effects caused by the drugs (which range from allergic problems to respiratory and gastrointestinal problems), increases the length of the patient's hospital stay and can compromise the health of the professionals involved in the treatment, which can considerably increase healthcare costs.

It was found that inguinal hernioplasty surgery is one of the most common procedures performed by surgeons, with an estimated 20 million hernioplasties per year worldwide. Inguinal hernia is characterized as one of the most common pathological conditions in adults, with the main incidence in males. The treatment of inguinal hernias is most often surgical and can cause localized pain of an acute and continuous nature (which can become chronic), leading to disability and loss of functionality in the patient.

Transcutaneous electrical nerve stimulation (TENS) has recently emerged as one of the main treatment modalities for chronic pain after hernioplasty, due to its analgesic (non-pharmacological) effect, and because it is a quick, cheap, safe and non-invasive means of treatment. In addition, when compared to other methods of analgesia, TENS is the method with the fewest side effects.

The interest in developing this topic has coexisted with the increasing expenditure on analgesic drugs in the hospital network. This is not only happening in Brazil or in underdeveloped countries, but also in first world countries such as the United States and Spain, which are starting to run deficits in their public coffers.

Some evaluation techniques fit the profile of this work, because in addition to minimizing costs in the hospital system, they demonstrate the emergence of a new technology with less risk to the integrity of the patient, as well as offering satisfaction and comfort to the population that needs care.

The research was made possible with the authorization of the doctor responsible for the management of the Hospital Sâo Domingos Sàvio in January 2004 and as a result of participating in a research project in 2003, which facilitated access to the catalog of patients undergoing the surgery chosen for this work.

In view of all the good results that this electric current has been bringing to patients by lowering the pain threshold, the time has come to discuss the viability of the resource for the hospital in terms of cost reduction, thus proposing the benefits of TENS as a substitute for analgesic drugs, justifying this study. To this end, all the costs of the drug procedure and the application of TENS were compared, in addition to demonstrating other relevant factors, such as epidemiology, incidence, which drugs are used in the postoperative period of the surgery in question and the rates of hospital infection and adverse effects caused by the drugs.

Within this panorama, we analyzed the interrelationship between the health system's expenditure on medicines and the reduction in costs with transcutaneous electrical nerve stimulation in patients undergoing inguinal hernioplasty surgery. All this will be discussed below.

The second chapter entitled Hospital management: quality, organization and costs in health services emphasizes quality in health services, analysis techniques to reduce costs, hospital organization and its singularities, and hospital costs in the public service. The third section deals with hospital-acquired infections due to the use of drugs with needles, subdivided into hospital-acquired infections in the context of health policies in Brazil and accidents at work involving sharps and health risks.

The fourth chapter deals with inguinal hernioplasty, defining the concept, incidence, treatment of inguinal hernia and noxious stimulation after surgical injury. The fifth chapter is related to the concept, application in inguinal hernia and the benefits of transcutaneous electrical nerve stimulation in the post-surgical period of inguinal hernioplasty. The sixth chapter describes the methodological procedures and materials used for this course conclusion. The seventh chapter reports the results, using graphs and simple statistics, and is made up of a discussion of the subjects covered in this monograph. Subsequently, the conclusion and the bibliographical reference will be found, finalizing this work and the academic activities.

Capitulo 2 HOSPITAL MANAGEMENT: QUALITY, ORGANIZATION AND COSTS IN HEALTH SERVICES

FLAVIA DIANA SANTOS FIGUEREDO; MILENA DE JESUS DA SILVA; HELDER HENRIQUE GOMES DA SILVA

2.1 Quality in health services

Quality in healthcare is one of the major obstacles to modern hospital management, which calls for not only good administration, but also proper organization and management, with the aim of reducing costs in healthcare services. In recent decades and in several countries, there has been a growing mobilization around the application of quality programs in hospital institutions with the aim of increasing their management and improving the efficiency of these services.

The health sector reform adopted a set of actions aimed at reducing health care costs. To this end, the governments of several countries have, among other measures, encouraged competition between hospitals, limited the total payment of bills, encouraged better management of health organizations through quality programs, limited procedures and access to more susceptible population subgroups and, finally, diverted some expenses to users.

Within this context, official instruments for evaluating the performance of hospital organizations in the Unified Health System have been developed in Brazil for some years, using a set of criteria that must be met on the basis of pre-established standards, based on the application of total quality concepts and techniques. A similar phenomenon can be observed in hospitals in the supplementary private network, which use certifications issued by internationally recognized assessment organizations as a market differentiator, demonstrating a growing concern with quality.

Nowadays, the adoption of quality programs in the health sector has arisen out of a concern to reduce the ever-increasing costs of hospital care when compared to total health expenditure. Every evaluation and formulation of quality programs is based on comparing an existing treatment with proven efficiency, such as pharmacotherapy, with a treatment that brings innovative options, with the aim of presenting not only efficiency and benefit for the patient, but also cost reduction and more favorable effects for the economy. From a clinical perspective, the use of a technology is justified if its effectiveness, or at least its efficiency, is positive. However, the economic point of view turns to efficiency.

Thinking in terms of efficiency implies considering the effectiveness of a process in relation to the resources that are required. The reason for this is that resources are limited in their possible applications, so the fewer resources needed to achieve a certain objective, the better, as this would leave more resources available to be used for other health purposes.

In the hospital sector, there is a lot of resistance to quality programs due to doctors, who have historically held power within these organizations and don't agree with the idea of cost containment, nor an evaluation of their work from the perspective of measuring quality, because they feel supervised and are afraid of losing their autonomy in the clinical management of patients. There are also financial sectors that do not attract the participation of the medical profession in this process. Doctors are mostly paid for the production of services and do not want to use their working hours for programs of this nature.

In addition, medical training is still based on the Flexnerian model, which emphasizes the clinical in its biological dimension and in which social, political and administrative aspects take a back seat. These issues are little observed in the curricula of medical schools, which is why there are obstacles to doctors' adherence to quality programs, due to deficiencies and limitations in their training.

2.2 Cost reduction analysis techniques

Economic analysis consists of determining the effects that should follow each of the possible options or subsequent courses of action in the election situation and comparing the options in terms of their social efficiency, i.e. their contribution to improving the well-being of people in society. In theory, this process is reflected in the studies that, in order to determine well-being, social costs and benefits must be taken into account.

There is a set of terms that must be assimilated in order to carry out an adequate approach to a good economic evaluation, which are: efficiency, effectiveness and availability. Efficiency is the benefit or usefulness of a technology for patients in a given population. It is based on the results of clinical trials, i.e. whether the new technology really works. Effectiveness means the results for the population it is aimed at and, finally, availability, which shows whether the new technology is accessible to those patients who could benefit from the product.

Analysis techniques for hospital economic evaluation usually fall into four categories: Cost-Decrease Analysis, Cost-Benefit Analysis, Cost-Effectiveness Analysis and Cost-Utility Analysis. These categories differ in the way they measure the effects of the options evaluated on health.

Cost-benefit analysis is called the original technique of economic evaluation. Basically, it is an accounting of costs and results in monetary terms, i.e. it is applied to determine the usefulness and economic viability of the new technology, relating the costs and benefits of the project for both the patients and the hospital, always expressed in financial terms. The main advantage of this approach is the comparison of an existing project with a new option, thus allowing the economic and health benefits to be compared.

Cost-effectiveness analysis is most commonly used in the health sector. It involves identifying and quantifying the costs and results of various alternative options or procedures to achieve the same objective, where the costs are expressed in financial terms and the consequences in physical and natural units.

Cost reduction analysis is a limited form of economic evaluation in which only the cost reduction in each sector is compared, while the other objectives achieved are not important and may or may not improve patient health.

Finally, cost-utility analysis makes it possible to compare different health interventions and outcomes in monetary terms and the health effects expressed in quality-adjusted life years or any other measure that uses the pathology-free life year as the unit of measurement.

The practical application of these techniques is based on the principle that the patient should receive the necessary attention to maintain their health and, furthermore, this analysis technique should be oriented towards the development of studies that make it possible to follow this principle through efficiency and rationality in the use of drugs.

The profile of this work fits in with the techniques of cost-benefit and cost-effectiveness analysis, as these are techniques that not only aim to reduce costs in the hospital system, but also demonstrate the emergence of a new technology with good results for the patient, bringing greater satisfaction and comfort to the population that needs care.

2.3 The hospital organization and its singularities

Hospital organization has changed over the centuries. From the concept of religiosity and intended for the population, it became an instrument of the therapeutic-curative and investigative medical practice that marked the birth of the clinic and reached the modern concept of the 19th century. In the second half of the 20th century, from the post-war period onwards, there was an increase in the use of hospitals, which had to improve their structure and the number of beds, becoming a central concern of national health systems.

Nowadays, the hospital environment is one of the most complex, not only because of its mission, but above all because it has a multidisciplinary team with a high degree of autonomy to provide preventive, curative and rehabilitative health care to inpatients, where routine technology is used. It is also a space for teaching-learning practice and scientific production.

As a company where the customer is the patient, there are some specific economic and organizational characteristics in hospitals that could be obstacles to the introduction of quality programs, for example, the laws of the market do not apply well to the sector in view of human needs and non-market priorities, which are imposed independently of production costs, market value and prices. In addition, competition is not a strong element in the environment of these organizations, as this is a chronically underserved segment in some countries, the variability of care demanded is enormous and each patient behaves subjectively differently, which makes it difficult to rigidly standardize health work processes and rationalize the supply of services.

There is also no symmetry of information in this market, as customers are generally lay people and don't have the ability to judge whether their treatment or their needs have been well met, making it difficult for them to exercise their consumer choices, which are immediate to production and there is no time for prior quality control. Despite this, many hospitals are currently creating evaluation forms for their users, focusing on the search for quality in hospital care, but in addition to the problems mentioned above, there is still, in most cases, a "bias" which can influence the patient's response towards the hospital. In this context, the direct action of managers and leaders in implementing management processes or models with a focus on hospital quality is essential for the quality of hospital care.

Both public and private organizations, regardless of their nature, are subject to ethical and legal principles, which regulate the health sector in order to provide good care and respect for patients and government policies, placing hospitals in the face of a variety of divergent interests.

The interests of users, who demand assistance in a wide variety of ways; the interests of health workers, who seek their livelihood and good working conditions; the interests of shareholders, in the case of a private hospital, which aims to make a profit; the interests of the network of manufacturers and distributors of supplies; of insurance companies and health plans, which establish a commercial relationship with the hospital; and, finally, the formally constituted interests of hospital management and the government, which focus on technical objectives and achieving the programmatic goals of health policy.

2.4 Hospital costs in the public service

2.4.1 Unified Health System and its guidelines

Before discussing hospital costs, it's important to know how the Unified Health Service (SUS) works. Since health is a right of every citizen, enshrined in the Federal Constitution in 1988, it is up to the State to provide the necessary conditions for this right to be enjoyed. This right is guaranteed by the public authorities at federal, state and municipal level, through policies aimed at reducing the risk of disease and enabling the implementation of actions and services for the promotion, protection and recovery of health.

The Union, the States, the Federal District and the Municipalities share responsibility for promoting coordination and interaction within the Unified Health System, ensuring universal and equal access to health actions and services. The SUS is a regionalized and hierarchical health system, which integrates all the health actions of the Union, States, Federal District and Municipalities, where each part fulfils specific functions and competencies, aiming at the reorganization and optimization of the care network of the Unified Health System, but articulated with each other, which characterizes the levels of management of the SUS in the three spheres of government.

Created by the 1988 Federal Constitution and regulated by Law No. 8080/90, known as the Organic Health Law, and Law No. 8141/90, the SUS has rules and regulations that govern the policies and actions in each Subsystem and states that it is necessary to involve the community in the management of the System and intergovernmental transfers of financial resources. It allows foreign capital to enter the health sector, with the right to participate directly or indirectly in all services.

Under the terms of the legislation, society participates in planning and controlling the implementation of health actions and services. This participation takes place through the Health Councils, which are present in the Union, States and Municipalities. Federal Law No. 8.142/1990 guarantees the establishment of permanent and deliberative councils at federal, state and municipal level, with the capacity to evaluate and supervise health services and resources. The federal sphere, which is managed by the Ministry of Health, is responsible for formulating national health policies, planning, standardizing, evaluating and controlling the SUS at a national level, as well as financing health actions and services through the application and distribution of public funds collected; the state level, which is administered by the state health secretariat and is responsible for formulating state health policy, coordinating and planning the SUS at state level, financing health actions and services through the application and distribution of public funds collected; the municipal sphere, whose manager is the municipal health department, whose role is to formulate municipal health policy and provide health actions and services, financed with its own resources or transferred by the federal and/or state administrator of the SUS.

2.4.2 Pharmaceuticals as substantial portions and alternatives for reducing costs

The high increase in the costs of many health technologies around the world and the growing pressure to reduce the budget in most countries has led to the need for economic intervention in health. Spending on this system is growing as a percentage of the Gross Domestic Product in many countries. Among these costs, attention is increasingly being paid to those related to pharmaceutical spending.

In Brazil, it was only in the 1980s, when public funds became more scarce, that administrators began to focus on allocating resources to hospitals. Around 40% of health spending in Brazil goes on paying for hospitalizations, while examinations account for 20% and consultations, which is the individual's first care, only 18% (Revista Visao Saùde, 2016). Also according to information from ABRAMGE, based on ANS data, 44.8% was spent on hospital admissions, 32.6% on consultations, 17.1% on complementary exams and 5.5% on therapies such as speech therapy, psychology and others.

The production and consumption of medicines in the world is concentrated in the developed countries. These capitalist and former socialist countries produce 89% of the world's medicines. Studies comparing the consumption of medicines in developed countries with less developed countries show that the former account for 70% of the world's production of pharmaceutical products.

Countries with the greatest health needs often allocate an insufficient proportion of their funds to health, which is often accompanied by the irrational use of medicines. Underdeveloped countries spend a high percentage of 20 to 45% of their Gross Domestic Product (GDP) on pharmaceutical products, which can be explained by the fact that the product is generally imported. In particular, Latin American countries spend approximately 25% of their health budget on the purchase of medicines, while the developed countries of North America, Western Europe and Eastern Europe spend approximately 15% of their health budget on the purchase of medicines.

In developed countries, 60% of spending on medicines is financed by the state and the population has access to qualified care free of charge. In developing countries, where a large part of the population does not have access to good hospital care, there is an even greater need to contain costs, including spending on medicines and reducing hospitalization days, and to find additional sources of technology and professionals to make up for this significant shortfall.

The economic discourse in the area of health *has* existed for almost 30 years. International agencies, non-governmental organizations and health ministries in most countries include discussion of economic and financial implications or constraints as part of medical or technical topics. Unfortunately, although the description and analysis contribute to raising awareness of the urgent need for the sector to be managed and organized with criteria of economic rationality, strategies and models that respond to the new international context are not always formulated. Furthermore, it is necessary to establish that the real objective of economics in this system is not just to describe and manipulate the sector's accounts and spending, but to guarantee equitable access to health care and maintenance.

The links between the economic system and health fulfill two main attributes: simultaneity and duality. Simultaneity refers to the fact that the population's health levels and the degree of economic development feed into each other, so it can be seen that a country cannot offer a high level of hospital support if it doesn't have a strong and stable economy. The term duality, on the other hand, is related to the well-being of the patient and, at the same time, minimizing economic costs, which means that it is necessary to offer good care and, at the same time, reduce the weight of the country's economic balance related to hospital and health costs in general.

As a whole, it is estimated that the cost of medicines represents a more than substantial portion of hospital expenses. Various authors list percentages of between 5 and 50%. The variation may be related to the type of service, level of care and the quality of decision-making processes and the information system involving medicines. In Spain, spending on medicines has risen above inflation in recent years, which jeopardizes the equitable provision of health care. In the United States, an increase in prices has been diagnosed along with the entry of new and expensive therapeutic agents, the highest annual health costs in individuals classified as physically inactive. In Peru, spending on medicines represents between 30 and 50% of the total invested in health, and these resources are generally insufficient to cover the demand from the public sector.

In order for costs to fall, it is necessary to look for the technological and professional, related and financial capacities needed to stand out in terms of relative performance without losing quality and efficiency. The challenge is to find a differentiation strategy that involves relatively lower costs, reducing them and freeing them up for other activities. For example, reforms have been proposed in the public health sector in Georgia and in the pharmaceutical sector in the *"newly independent states"* (Armenia, Azerbaijan, the Republic of Moldova, the Russian Federation, Ukraine, among others) with the aim of increasing access to health services for the neediest populations.

One of the most notable features of the cost-based strategic management model is the exploitation of diversity, as it teaches you to accept the possibility of abandoning ownership of a technology or piece of equipment in order to concentrate on studying alternative forms and types of service that can enhance the service and, at the same time, be useful to users. To illustrate the point, in the period between 2009 and 2012, Brazil reduced its purchase price by 30%.

Capitulo 3 HOSPITAL-ACQUIRED INFECTIONS DUE TO THE USE OF NEEDLES IN THE APPLICATION OF DRUGS

MATEUS LIMA SANTOS; SUYANE CAROLINE FEITOSA DE\ SANTANA; VANESSA OLIVEIRA BARBOSA

3.1 Hospital infections in the context of health policies in Brazil

A hospital-acquired infection (HAI) is one that the healthcare professional acquires after admitting the patient and which can manifest itself with symptoms during hospitalization or after the patient has been discharged, i.e. when it is related to hospitalization or hospital procedures, it can be classified as a hospital-acquired infection.

This type of infection has a high hospital mortality rate worldwide, the most recurrent of which are linked to the central venous catheter, most of which are associated with the bloodstream, which occurs when the micro-organism present at the catheter insertion site falls into the bloodstream and thus causes an infection with serious clinical compromise. Intravascular catheters, especially venous catheters, are widely used in intensive care to administer medication, hydroelectrolyte solutions, blood and also to monitor physiological patterns. With their presence in the deep venous system, the risk of infection is high.

This problem is growing progressively all over the world and is considered a significant public health problem. In Brazil, the average hospital infection rate is around 15%, while in the USA and Europe it is 10%. The main factors behind these percentages are: immune status; age (newborns and the elderly are more vulnerable); abuse of antibiotics; medical procedures, especially invasive ones, and immunosuppression.

The process of patient safety goes through several stages, from how medicines are prescribed, dispensed, administered and monitored in healthcare facilities. The better prepared healthcare professionals are, the less likely errors are to occur (PAIM et al, 2016). Medication administration errors are highly significant, accounting for around 19.4% of all adverse events.

Primary bloodstream infections related to short-term central venous catheters represent a high cost for hospital organizations. Evaluating the quality of hospital infection control programs pointed to the need for better structuring of infection control services, especially those related to health care. Knowing the real financial impact of hospital-acquired infections can contribute to the search for preventive actions to reduce hospital-acquired infection rates, so that not only do healthcare professionals have more job security, but hospitals don't have to spend more.

The costs of hospital infections are divided into direct, indirect or preventive and immeasurable. The former represent the costs of diagnosis, examinations and treatment of the infected patient, which includes medication, additional days and precautionary measures. Indirect or preventive costs correspond to investments to avoid, reduce and control hospital infections. There are also the immeasurable costs, which are the pain and suffering of the patient and their family, which affect their quality of life; they can result in the inactivity of a limb, the loss of function of an organ or even death related to hospital infections.

3.2 Accidents at work with sharps and health risks

Among health professionals, those most at risk from sharp materials are nurses. Biological risks are related to the professional's contact with microorganisms, contagious infectious material, exposure to blood and organic fluids. Biological risks in health services are directly related to mechanical risks, which refer to injuries caused by falls, handling sharp or penetrating objects, these risks are mainly related to procedures for contact with body fluids, sneezing or splashing and proper handling of sharps, with disposal in a rigid and appropriate box, without attempts to reattach, remove or break the needle.

In relation to sharps, there are occupational risks related to the handling of waste contaminated with biological material: hepatitis B with a risk of around 30%; hepatitis C, 3%; AIDS, transmitted by the HIV virus, with a risk of 0.3%.

Among the main infections to which healthcare workers are subject are pulmonary tuberculosis, cytomegalovirus (CMV virus infection), viral hepatitis, Human Immunodeficiency Virus (HIV) infection and Acquired Immunodeficiency Syndrome (AIDS). These are now considered worldwide to be the main biological risks for health workers. Taking into account the most recurrent accidents, contusions were the most frequent injuries, making up 31.91% of the events, while those caused by piercing and cutting, broken glass, scalpel blades, razors and needles were in second place, with an index of 27.66%. This clearly shows that there is still no special attention paid to accidents involving sharps. The large number of accidents involving sharps is the result of a lack of awareness on the part of health professionals about how to handle them so as to ensure greater safety.

The majority of accidents occurred among female professionals (84.2%). The professional category most affected was nursing technicians (42.1%). Percutaneous exposure was the most common, with 84.2%. The majority of accidents were caused by 3 needles, corroborating the findings which also identified blood as the most reported biological material, with 86.3% of accidents.

In this respect, the activity of nursing care takes place in person and uninterruptedly, for better information involving hygiene tasks, the administration of medicines, the handling and preparation of surgical instruments, as well as the handling of contaminated excretions.

After exposure to accidents at work, the psychological factor suffers from the doubts and uncertainties of the consequences of the accident. The experience of having an accident involving biological material causes different feelings among professionals, but the main feelings expressed by professionals are fear, anguish, anxiety, nervousness and despair related to the possibility of being infected with a virus such as HIV, which will lead to changes in their daily lives. The psychological stress experienced as a result of a percutaneous accident can have psychosocial repercussions, leading to changes in social, family and professional relationships.

Capitulo 4 INGUINAL HERNIOPLASTY: CONCEPTS AND ACUTE POSTOPERATIVE PAIN

DARLEN MILENA DE OLIVEIRA SANTOS; HANNA BEATRIZ DE MELO MORAES E SILVA; ISABELA DE ALMEIDA ROCHA

4.1 Concept and incidence of inguinal hernia

Hernias are the total or partial protrusion of an organ contained in a peritoneal lining outside the abdominal wall due to malformation or muscle-aponeurotic weakening. They can occur in various positions: umbilical, around the navel (10%), epigastric, in the midline of the abdomen (6%), incisional, in the region of a scar (10%), femoral, by the displacement of part of the intestine to the thigh (5%) or inguinal, in the region of the groin (69%).

A hernia (Latin, disruption; Greek, sprout) is defined as the protrusion of an organ through an opening in the protective tissue layers of the internal abdominal organs. The most common cause of abdominal wall hernias is major local surgery.

Inguinal hernias are the most common (75%), affecting approximately 1.5% of the general population and 5% of the male population.

The higher prevalence in males is partly due to the size of the spermatic cord, which is much larger than the round ligament, and the testicular vaginal process is often less obliterated than the corresponding female canal of Nuck. In women, the external inguinal ring is smaller, and the aponeurosis of the external oblique muscle that covers the inguinal canal is stronger. Men have a constitutional predisposition to both direct and indirect inguinal hernias and women are more likely than men to report post-operative pain.

The inguinal hernia is one of the most frequent diagnoses to predispose to pediatric surgery, with a prevalence of 0.8 - 4.4%. This is because the inguinal canal develops as the child grows, and they still have weak abdominal muscles.

In this way, inguinal hernia repair is one of the most frequently performed pediatric surgical methods, and it is estimated that only 25-50% may be responsible for the appearance of future hernias. Hernia recurrence is a complication of hernia correction, although it occurs less frequently in children than in adults.

In females, the layers of the vaginal processes normally fuse together, closing off the entrance to the inguinal canal in the abdominal cavity. In some individuals these processes remain open and this failure of fusion can result in an inguinal hernia.

In males, the process of testicular descent normally takes place during the seventh month of pregnancy, when the testicle crosses the inguinal canal following the peritoneal sac of the vaginal process. Completion of the descent and fixation take place between the seventh and ninth month of pregnancy, after the patent vaginal process has normally closed. Failure to close usually leads to a hernia.

Around 1 to 4% of male neonates are affected, with 60% of hernias occurring on the right, 30% on the left and the rest bilateral. Usually, this is not a difficult clinical diagnosis to make and the parents observe a reddish bulge in the inguinal region which, when touched, the child reports as painful.

4.2 Treatment and noxious stimulation after inguinal hernia surgery

Hernias are only treated surgically, by means of hernioplasty. There are numerous techniques for the surgical repair of abdominal wall defects and they have evolved in recent years. Basically, they are divided into techniques using only primary aponeurotic sutures - which must be tension-free - and techniques using synthetic prostheses (meshes). The repair of inguinal hernias performed using a meshless and tension-free surgical method is widely used and has become increasingly popular with surgeons. Numerous studies show that techniques using the patient's own tissue for hernia repair have a recurrence rate of 10 to 50%, while the use of prostheses restricts recurrence to 3 to 17%.

Inguinal hernioplasty surgeries are quite common and performed frequently in Brazilian hospitals, and are the fifth most common surgery performed in hospitals in Rio de Janeiro.

Despite the high frequency of surgical repair, surgeons still don't achieve perfect results and the rate of surgical failure (recurrence) is still significant. Hernias are among the diseases that have affected men for the longest time, and are one of the first diseases to be detected due to their easily identifiable clinical signs. The concept of tension-free hernioplasty is commonly used because this method uses a synthetic mesh, as it is an easier technique, generates less post-operative pain, heals quickly and can be performed under local anesthesia.

In view of the hernioplasty techniques without mesh, the Shouldice technique is currently considered the gold standard for this case. Compared to the other techniques, it has a lower chance of recurrence, with a recurrence rate of 5%. The choice of whether or not to use a mesh prosthesis depends very much on the patient's age and the type of hernia. Direct or mixed hernias have a higher risk of recurrence due to the weakness of the tissue, justifying the use of mesh.

The severity of pain is not directly proportional to the amount of damaged tissue or the severity of the injury. Many factors can influence the perception of this symptom, such as fatigue, depression, anger, fear, anxiety about the disease, feelings of hopelessness and helplessness, which leads us to understand that in addition to the physical component, the mental component is also present in the appearance or worsening of symptoms. Faced with the vast possibility of causes, the use of painkillers is only a fraction of the care needed to understand all areas of pain. Because it is common after surgical procedures, pain has been seen as something natural that comes from this type of procedure, despite being the symptom that bothers most, it is left aside in the face of other complications such as fistulas, bleeding and others.

Pain must be assessed accurately and regularly so that treatment is always appropriate to improve the patient's symptoms. Antalgic therapy should combine two or more peripheral or central analgesic techniques, both preventively and in the postoperative period with and without complications; including the use of non-pharmacological methods, allowing for fewer drugs and consequently minimizing side effects and costs.

Post-operative pain is one of the main problems of hernioplasty, generating great concern because there is a high incidence of chronic post-operative pain in patients; this directly affects quality of life, delaying ambulation and hindering the chances of patients being discharged from hospital early, thus explaining the emergence of concern about effective multimodal treatment. Studies have reported greater chronic post-operative pain in patients treated with the Liechtenstein technique. Others have described that the laparoscopic method reduces the occurrence of acute pain and edema in the postoperative period, allowing patients to return to their daily activities more quickly.

Pain in the inguinal region after herniorrhaphy is a common symptom. In the first 24 hours, it subsides with the use of analgesics, decreases progressively and disappears after a few weeks. Some patients after undergoing the herniorrhaphy procedure complain of pain that makes it impossible for them to return to their normal activities.

Studies have shown that pain is one of the body's protective mechanisms and occurs whenever any tissue is being damaged, causing the individual to react and thus eliminate the painful stimulus. According to Bishop (1984), the gate theory states that fibers from the skin, viscera and other structures converge on the transmission cells, resulting in both facilitating and inhibiting output from these cells. Pain associated with peripheral nerve damage is characterized by hyperalgesia and hyperesthesia attributable to excessive release of the pain pathway.

Capitulo 5 TRANSCUTANEOUS ELECTRICAL NERVE STIMULATION IN INGUINAL HERNIA

MILENA DE JESUS DA SILVA; VICTÓRIA ÂNDERSEN DA SLVA RODRIGUES; LiCIA SANTOS OLIVEIRA

5.1 History and concept of TENS

Electricity has been used to relieve pain for thousands of years and was first studied by Aristotle. In the mid-1800s and early 1900s, several physicists and dentists reported the use of electricity as an analgesic and anesthetic. However, electrical stimulation for pain relief was not fully accepted by the medical profession until Wall and Sweet published their theory of pain gates in 1967.

Transcutaneous electrical nerve stimulation (TENS) is an easily applicable, non-invasive mechanism that can be applied to various age groups for analgesia purposes. This device is low cost, free of adverse effects and has few contraindications. There are various theories proposed for the mechanism of analgesia acquired by TENS, the main one being based on the behavioral theory proposed by Melzack and Wall in 1965. This theory has the operation of the descending inhibitory pain system, in which the activity of the pain transmission neurons is located in the dorsal horn of the medulla and generates electro cortical effects in the sensory motor cortex.

Clinically, TENS is used at various frequencies, intensities and pulse widths. It is a device with a bidirectional, non-ionizing and asymmetrical current that can alternate from 1 to 250 Hz (hertz). The stimulation frequency is classified as high-frequency (conventional), low-frequency (acupuncture), burst, and brief-intense, which implies different analgesic mechanisms. The intensity is determined by the patient, either on a sensory or motor level, depending on the parameters used.

At the sensory level, the intensity is increased until the patient feels a tingling or "prickling" sensation on the skin without motor contraction. At the motor level, the intensity is increased until there is a muscle contraction. Normally, this stimulation is increased to the maximum without being harmful to the patient. In general, high-frequency TENS is applied at low intensities and is characterized as conventional TENS. In contrast, low-frequency TENS is applied at high intensities, resulting in motor contraction; this mode of stimulation is called acupuncture TENS.

5.2 The benefits of applying and using TENS compared to analgesics in inguinal hernias

The following procedures are recommended for the treatment of post-surgical pain: opioids, non-steroidal anti-inflammatory drugs, local anesthetics or sedatives, all of which can promote unsatisfactory analgesia accompanied by adverse effects. The second most abused drug is narcotic medication, which is used for post-operative or pre-operative pain. In 2003, there was an increase in unpremeditated (overdose) deaths related to the use of opioid analgesics, due to dose abuse.

In North Carolina (United States) in 2000, it was observed that the cost of medication per patient in the post-operative period of lower abdominal surgery was around R$176.00, of which R$173.00 was for non-steroidal anti-inflammatory drugs.

Nowadays, there is a great tendency to reduce the use of drugs due to their considerable side effects, such as gastro-intestinal (nausea and vomiting), allergic skin effects, respiratory depression, confusion and agitation and urinary retention. Around 29% of adverse effects are associated with the use of analgesics. Globally, the costs of side effects are very high, ranging from 67 to 114 billion reais per year in the United States. The costs of adverse effects associated with opioids used in surgical patients exceed R$ 51,220.00 per year and increase hospital stays by approximately one and a half days, representing an additional cost of R$ 3,309.60 per patient.

At *LDS Hospital* (*Salt Lake City*, *Utah* - United States), adverse effects are responsible for an increase of R$ 500.38 when only one clinical manifestation is present and an increase of R$ 4,668.90 when there is more than one manifestation. The clinical changes in side effects that most increased hospital costs in terms of days of hospitalization and drugs used were: confusion and agitation, representing an increase of R$ 3,711.48; urinary retention, with an increase of R$ 3.061.38; respiratory depression, with a cost of R$ 2,466.44; gastrointestinal manifestations, representing an expense of R$ 2,009.40; and last but not least, allergic skin effects, representing an amount of R$ 823.46.

With this in mind, transcutaneous electrical nerve stimulation (TENS) has been proposed as an alternative therapy for the treatment of post-operative pain, as it has the advantages of being easy to apply and has no side-effects or side-effects, as well as being a non-invasive, safe and easy-to-apply technique, which also helps to reduce the risk of hospital-acquired infections.

According to recent studies, TENS has reduced morphine requirements by 61% in the treatment of lower abdominal postoperative pain. This reduction in drug doses means that the rates of adverse effects caused by the drugs fall and that the risk of hospital-acquired also decreases, minimizing the patient's hospital stay.

It was concluded that conventional high-frequency, low pulse width TENS reduced the perception of pain stimulation during the postoperative period of inguinal hernioplasty in the patients in this study, statistically eliminating the need to administer analgesic drugs, as shown in graph 01.

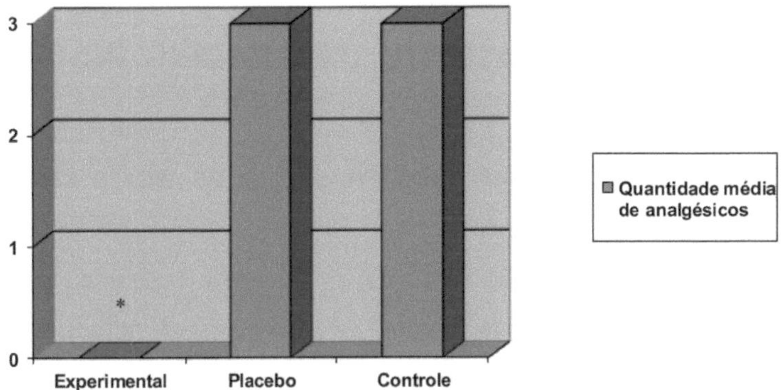

Graph 01: Comparative analysis of the quantity of analgesic drugs administered in the experimental, placebo and control groups (* $p<0.05$).

Capitulo 6 EVALUATION OF HOSPITAL COST REDUCTION THROUGH TENSING IN PATIENTS UNDERGOING INGUINAL HERNIOPLASTY

ISABELA DE ALMEIDA ROCHA; HALLYSON FRANKLINN DE WETTE SANTOS; PAULO AUTRAN LEITE LIMA

The results of TENS related to the reduction of the pain threshold and the reduction in the number of drugs requested by patients were obtained from the research by Melo; Santana Filho (2003) represented by one of the extensions of the same research project as this study, whose name was the use of conventional high-frequency TENS and low pulse width in the analgesic requirement of the immediate postoperative period of inguinal hernia surgery.

The drugs used in the postoperative period of inguinal hernioplasty surgery, the ages and sexes of the patients were recorded in the medical records. In addition, the months of research, the average number of drugs administered and the total number of surgical procedures were organized using a form of our own design.

Patients ranging in age from 1 month to 80 years were catalogued from June 2016 to May 2017 and analyzed by gender, age group (0-11, 12-18, 19-59, 6080) and cases of inguinal hernia during the month.

The total cost analysis of the applications of the drugs *Cataflam*, *Novalgina* and *Voltaren,* together with the total cost analysis of the TENS applications, was carried out using simple descriptive statistics and shown in graphs (pie charts, columns and rows).

6.1 Flow of patients undergoing inguinal hernioplasty

The demand for patients undergoing inguinal hernioplasty at the hospital studied reached a total of 382 between the months of June 2016 to 5.33 standard. As shown in graph 02.

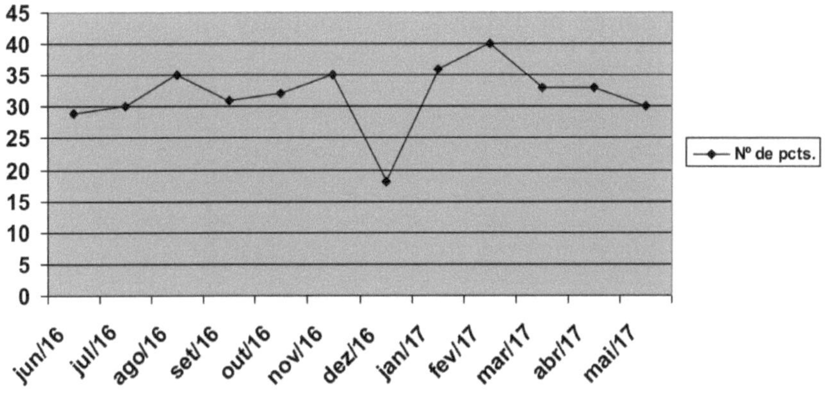

Graph 02: Incidence of patients undergoing inguinal hernia surgery per month.

Source: Produced by the authors.

May 2017, totaling one year of care for this pathology.

This resulted in an average of 31.83 surgeries per month, with a deviation. This flow of patients varies according to the hospital's capacity and the number of inhabitants in the region. The hospital we analyzed performs around 27 surgeries a day and has 73 beds to cater for different types of pathologies and people of all ages. In larger hospitals and in cities with a large population, this demand could be substantially higher.

The months of January and February saw the highest concentrations of these surgeries (36 and 40, respectively), while December saw the lowest number (18). This is explained by the fact that in the last month of the year, the hospital takes doctors on vacation. As a result, patients who would have undergone inguinal hernia surgery in December are scheduled for the following two months.

6.2 Sex-related cases of inguinal hernioplasty

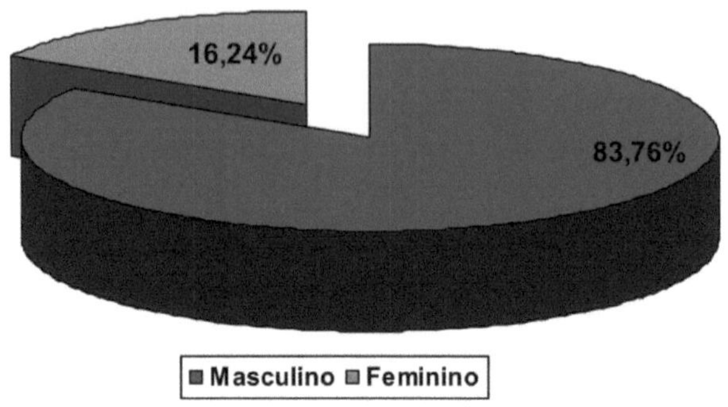

Graph 03: Incidence of patients undergoing inguinal hernia surgery by gender. **Source**: Produced by the authors.

The incidence of male patients undergoing inguinal hernioplasty is higher than the opposite sex, reaching 83.76% (320 patients) of cases, while the female sex represents a population of only 16.24% (62 patients), as can be seen in the following graph.

This study corroborates Ponka (1980), who reported a high percentage for males (93.3%). This high incidence in men is explained by the fact that the transverse fascia is firmer and more resistant in women. In addition, other important factors such as the type of activity carried out at work, impaired abdominal muscle tone with advancing age and inadequate exercise are reported as conditions that increase intra-abdominal pressure and can cause inguinal hernias, as stated by Bervilacqua (1988) and Mullins (2004).

6.3 Age-related cases of inguinal hernioplasty

The highest incidence of patients undergoing inguinal hernioplasty was in the 19-59 age group, with 195 cases, followed by the 0-11 age group with 114, the 60-80 age group with 55 and finally the 12-18 age group with 18, as can be seen in graph 04.

This higher incidence in the 19-60 age group is explained by the studies of

Ajabnoor et al (1992), Rodrigues; Guimaraes (1997) and Read (1998) that with advancing age the natural process of aging and weakening of the aponeurotic and muscular fascial structures is progressive and can be associated with conditions that increase intra-abdominal pressure, i.e. it is in this age group that people are at their most productive in their jobs and some of them make manual efforts with heavy loads, facilitating the origin of inguinal hernias.

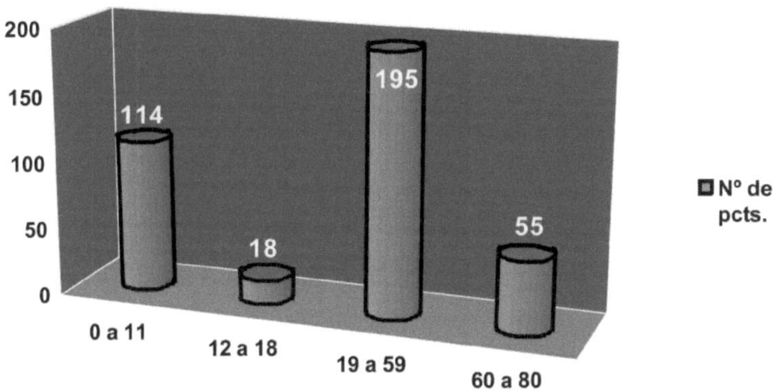

Graph 04: Incidence of patients undergoing inguinal hernia surgery by age group. Source: Produced by the authors.

With regard to the 0-11 age group, Collins (2002) found that the incidence of inguinal hernias is due to problems in embryonic development, affecting children of both sexes, with the most common surgical problem being among neonates. Finally, no data was found in the literature that could explain the low incidence in the 12-18 age group.

6.4 Inguinal hernioplasty cases related to age group and sex

The male sex was higher than the opposite sex in all age groups, which proves the greater impact on this sex. It can also be seen that in males the highest incidence was found in the 19-59 age group (170 cases), as this is related to the physiological and work-related conditions already explained. In second place was the 0-11 age group, with 83 cases. As shown in Graph 05.

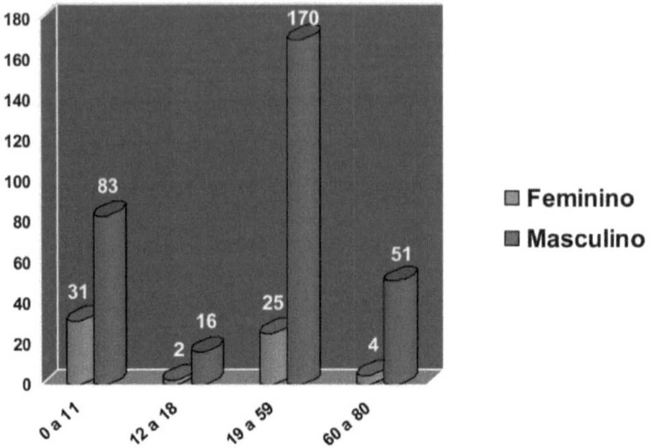

Graph 05: Incidence of patients undergoing inguinal hernia surgery by age group and gender.

Source: Produced by the authors.

According to Collins (2002) and Hebra (2004), the occurrence of hernias between the ages of 0-11 can be explained by a defective embryonic process of testicular formation, i.e. after testicular descent the vaginal process normally closes, but in pathological cases this process does not fuse, leading to the formation of a hernia.

In females, the highest incidence was in the 011 age group (31 cases), which can be explained by the studies of Donn; Faix (1994) and Collins (2002), who also report embryonic problems in the vaginal processes, which do not fuse and become continuously open, potentially causing an inguinal hernia. In second place was the 19-59 age group, which can be explained by the type of work or effort carried out, according to Hebra (2004).

6.5 Cost analysis between drugs and TENS

The overall annual cost of medicines (R$3,438.50) was much higher than the overall annual cost of TENS (R$424.06) for inguinal hernia surgery. As a result, there was a reduction in costs of R$3,014.44, as shown in Graph 06. This amount could be reverted to other areas of health that need more investment and technology, as reported by Luiza; Castros; Nunes (1999) and

Artmann; Rivera (2003).

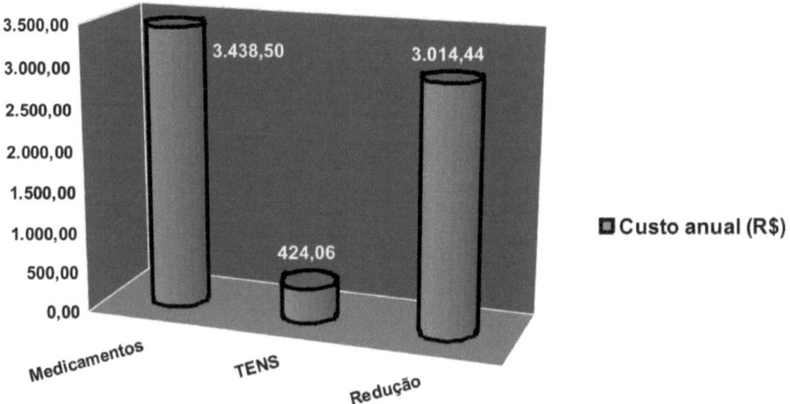

Graph 06 - Annual cost in R$ for inguinal hernia surgery.

Source: Produced by the authors.

The R$3,438.50 spent on pharmaceuticals includes three types of medicine (*Cataflam*, *Voltaren* and *Novalgina*), cotton wool, alcohol, a needle and a syringe. The following materials and their respective prices are used for each application of *Cataflam*: a 75mg ampoule (R$1.25), a cotton ball (R$0.01), 5mL of 70% alcohol (R$0.25) and a 5mL syringe[*1] (R$0.50).

Thus, each dose costs R$2.01. In the case of *Voltaren*, the following are used: an ampoule (R$1.31), a cotton ball (R$0.01), 5mL of 70% alcohol (R$0.25) and a 5mL syringe[*1] (R$0.50). As a result, each application costs R$2.07. Finally, for each dose of *Novalgina, the following are* used: a 2mL ampoule (R$1.64), a cotton ball (R$0.01), 5mL of 70% alcohol (R$0.25) and a 10mL syringe[*1] (R$0.81), totaling R$2.71 per application.

In general, during one year of post-operative care for inguinal hernioplasty, 1454 doses of the drugs mentioned were administered, 452 of which were *Cataflam*, totaling R$908.52, 289 of *Voltaren,* costing R$598.23 and, finally,

---

*1 Each syringe comes with its own needle, which is included in the price in brackets.

*2 Average obtained through a random selection of students and teachers at the Tiradentes University Rehabilitation Center.

*3 KW/h was calculated according to the local energy operator's rate.

713 doses of *Novalgina, totaling* R$1,932.23.

Overall, each patient received an average of 3.80 doses. The individual averages of drugs administered were: *Novalgina* 1.86 doses, *Cataflam* 1.18 and *Voltaren* 0.75.

The R$424.06 spent on TENS includes: the equipment with 02 cables and 04 electrodes, gel, adhesive tape, paper towels and energy consumption. The Ibramed Neurodyn portable TENS device costs R$298.00, which is added to the total number of applications. Only one device meets the current needs of the hospital in question and the purchase of the device already includes 02 cables and 04 electrodes.

Each TENS application costs an average of 10g of gel[*2] (R$ 0.05), 87.6cm of adhesive tape[*2] (R$ 0.03), 04 sheets of paper towel[*2] (R$ 0.01) and KW/h (R$ 0.02)[*3] . According to Melo; Santana Filho (2003), according to the analogue pain ladder, 3 applications of 30 minutes each were enough for the patient to be discharged from hospital with zero pain. As a result, each patient would cost the hospital R$ 0.33.

During the period from June 2002 to May 2003, 382 inguinal hernioplasty surgeries were performed. If TENS were used in these procedures, the costs would amount to R$ 126.06 in applications, which added to the price of the device would total an annual cost of R$ 424.06.

It is important to note that the TENS device would only be an initial expense and could be used for several years, if properly maintained, further reducing costs in other years of care.

Since TENS is a non-invasive method, it represents a reduction in costs when it comes to hospital expenses related to hospital infections caused by needles.

These costs can be understood as direct and indirect costs, the direct costs occurring when the patient's stay in hospital is prolonged or when their return to the job market is delayed, and the indirect costs occurring when there are disorders that are difficult to assess, such as malaise and pain, according to the study by Silva (2003). Although the patient is the main target of the study, we must not forget the professionals who deal with the handling of sharps, who are currently exposed to contamination from the acquired immunodeficiency syndrome virus and hepatitis B and C, as stated by Marziele; Rodrigues (2002).

Another important point is that TENS has no adverse effects, unlike the drugs *Cataflam*, *Novalgina* and *Voltaren*. According to Melo (2000), the main side effects of Cataflam are gastrointestinal toxicity, nausea, fatigue and edema.

Novalgin, regardless of the dose, can cause hypersensitivity reactions in patients, with the main adverse effects being: fever, chills, sore throat, difficulty swallowing, inflammatory lesions in the mouth, nose and throat, nausea, shortness of breath, numbness, among others. Finally, *Voltaren* can cause abdominal pain, diarrhea, nausea and headache.

If the patient has any of these adverse effects, their day in hospital will be extended and new drugs will be administered to cure the condition. This would increase the hospital's costs and the risks to the patient's health, which could lead to unfavorable clinical conditions for early improvement. In addition, it is more advantageous to use TENS, because it is a non-invasive technique, it doesn't hurt and it doesn't cause side effects, providing well-being and satisfaction to the patient, reducing the time spent in hospital and, as a result, returning to social activity more quickly.

The techniques of cost-benefit and cost-effectiveness analysis fit into this work because, as mentioned above and proposed by Gonzalez (1999), they are hospital economic evaluation techniques that aim to reduce costs in addition to effective results for the treatment of patients and their well-being, with the main advantage of comparing an existing and usual procedure carried out by the hospital unit with a new option, allowing the comparison of its economic and health benefits.

Conventional TENS has been shown to reduce hospital costs when compared to analgesic drugs in the post-operative period of inguinal hernioplasty through a cost-benefit and cost-effectiveness analysis, which in addition to saving the hospital sector brings satisfaction and well-being to the patient. R$3,014.44 would be reduced in application costs alone, which could be redistributed to other areas lacking in medical and hospital resources. Not to mention the possible costs of side effects and hospital infections that could occur when a patient undergoes an invasive, pharmacological procedure.

It is worth noting that this theme does not end with this monograph, as studies will continue for the development of a proposal for a master's thesis.

The proposal for the master's degree is to apply TENS to other pathologies and use the data collected to see if there is an even greater reduction in the costs of the hospital system. It is hoped that this monograph has contributed to the formulation of new studies, further enhancing the field of administrative physiotherapy and hospital management.

As a suggestion for further work, other physiotherapeutic resources could be studied that are economically viable for the hospital and that reduce the patient's length of stay, making physiotherapy grow even more in the hospital environment.

REFERENCES

ALVES, E. M. S. et al. Transcutaneous electrical nerve stimulation for postCesarean section analgesia. Revista Dor, Sao Paulo, v. 16, n. 4, p.263-266, Oct. 2015. GN1 Genesis Network.

ALVES, M. M. et al. Hospital Infection Control as an Indicator for Quality in the Health Service. In: Proceedings of the Symposium on Active Methodologies: Innovations for teaching and learning in basic and higher education. Blucher Education Proceedings. v. 2, n. 1, p. 158-172. Sao Paulo: Blucher, 2017.

ARAUJO, M. J. D.; ARTMANN, E.; ANDRADE, M. A. C. Démarche Estratégica: an innovative and effective way of analyzing institutional mission. Physis: Revista de Saùde Coletiva. 2013, vol.23, n.2, pp.319-343.

ARAÙJO, I. M. M, OLIVEIRA, A. G. R.C. Interfaces between collective health and political ecology: vulnerability, territory and social metabolism. Rio de Janeiro, V. 41, N. Especial, P. 276-286, JUN 2017.

ARTMANN, E.; RIVERA, F. J. U. A demarche stratégique (strategic hospital management): an instrument for coordinating hospital practice based on opportunity costs and solidarity. Ciência & Saùde Coletiva, v.08, n.02, p. 497-499, 2003.

BARBOSA, M. C. M. et al. Biological risks and adherence to personal protective equipment: perception of hospital nursing staff. Rev Pesq Saùde, 17(2): 87-91, May-Aug, 2016.

BARROS, F. P. C.; FILHO, A. N. Universal health coverage. Cad. Saùde Pùblica, Rio de Janeiro, 31(6):1333-1335, jun, 2015.

BEVILACQUA, R. G. Manual de cirurgia. 2. ed. Sâo Paulo: EPU, 1998.

BISHOP, B. Pain: Its physiology and rationale If management neuroanatomical substrate of pain. Physical Therapy, v.64, p. 924, 1984.

BUENO, D. R. et al. The costs of physical inactivity in the world: a review study. Ciência & Saùde Coletiva, 21(4):1001-1010, 2016.

CARDOSO, I. L.; CUNHA, J. R. A. O minimo existencial do direito à saù no SUS: o caso do Programa Saùde da Familia. Journal of Ibero-American Health Law. Brasilia, 5(4):9-26, Oct./Dec, 2016.

CARDOSO, J. A.; BARRETO, W. L. The use of TENS and ultrasound in the conservative treatment of lateral epicondylitis of the elbow (tennis elbow). Caderno de ciências biológicas e da saùde: Boa vista, Roraima, n. 3, p.62-83, 2013.

CARRIEL, T. C.; CARDOSO, A. L. Risks of contamination by accidents at work with sharp materials in the health area. Rev. UNINGA, Maringà, v. 54, n. 1, p. 91-101, Oct./Dec. 2017.

CARVALHO, G. Public health in Brazil. Estudos Avançados, [s.l.], v. 27, n. 78, p.7-26, 2013. FapUNIFESP (SciELO).

COELHO FILHO, Sebastiâo Célio Horta et al. Importance of Primary Health Care in Medicine: Simultaneous Analysis of Two Colleges, under the Vision of Teachers and Students. Journal Of Biosciences And Medicines. n 5, p. 612. nov. 2017.

COLLINS, S. Hydrocele and hernia in children.Net. Louisiana, May 2002 Available at: <http://www.emedicine.com/ped/topic1037.htm>. Accessed on 01/05/2004.

CORREIO, A. K.; LEONICE, M. Calculating the costs of hospital medical procedures in Brazilian hospitals. Revista de Administraçâo Hospitalar, v.11, n.1, pp. 1-11, January/March, 2014.

COSTA, G. P. C. Preventive civil liability: Analysis of the institute applied to the provision of services by private hospitals. 2017. 62f. Master's dissertation - Federal University of Uberlândia. 2017.

CRUZ, M. F. et al. Simultaneity of risk factors for chronic non-communicable diseases among elderly people in the urban area of Pelotas, Rio Grande do Sul, Brazil. Cad. Saùde Pùblica 2017; 33(2):e00021916.

CUNHA, J. D. S; GOMES, R. N S. Risks of accidents with sharps in nursing professionals: integrative literature review. ReonFacema. 2017 Apr-Jun; 3(2):499-505.

DALTON, R. N. et al. Clinical Economics: Calculating the cost of acute postoperative pain medication. Journal of Pain and Symptom Management, v.19, n.4, p. 295-308, 2000.

DANSKI, M. T. R.; et al. Costs of central venous catheter-related infection in adults: a systematic review. Rev baiana Enferm. 2017;31(3);e22079.

DEUS, A. R. Quality in health care - a look at the literature. National Congress of Excellence in Management, 2016.

DONN, S. M.; FAIX, R. G. Neonatal emergencies. Rio de Janeiro: Revinter, 1994.

EIDY, M. et al. Preemptive Analgesic Effects of Transcutaneous Electrical Nerve Stimulation (TENS) on Postoperative Pain: A Randomized, DoubleBlind, Placebo-Controlled Trial. Iranian Red Crescent Medical Journal. 2016; 18(4)

ELAHI, F. et al. Ultrasound guided peripheral nerve stimulation implant for management of intractable pain after inguinal herniorrhaphy. Pain Physician Journal 18:E31- E38, 2015

FEBRAFAR. (May 01, 2017). 2017 DRUG READJUSTMENT SET. Source: Brazilian Federation of Associative and Independent Pharmacy Networks.

FERNANDES, M. A.; SILVA, J. S. Feelings and emotions of nursing workers in the face of accidents at work: an integrative review. Rev Pre Infec e Saùde.2017;3(2):45-52.

FERREIRA, J. R.; et al. International cooperation in health: the case of

Fiocruz. História, Ciências, Saùde - Manguinhos, Rio de Janeiro, v.23, n.2, abr.-jun. 2016, p.267-276.

GARCIA, L. P. et al. Expenditure of Brazilian families on medicines according to family income: analysis of the 2002-2003 and 2008-2009 Family Budget Survey. Cad. Saùde Pùblica, Rio de Janeiro, v. 29, n. 8, p. 1605-1616, Aug. 2013 .

GONZALEZ, A. M. G. La farmacoeconomia en la eficiencia de la salud pùblica. Revista Cubana Salud Pùblica, v.25, n.01, p. 81-5, 1999.

GONÇALVES, M.; ALEMÂO, M. M.; DRUMOND, H. A. Study of the use of cost information as a management tool in a public organization: The study of SIGHCustos. Perspectives on Management & Knowledge, v. 3, p. 210-226, 2013.

GONÇALVES, M. A. et al. Health financing and the relevance of cost information in the public health sector: study of the cost knowledge base of the Hospital Foundation of the State of Minas Gerais - FHEMIG. In: XXII CONGRESSO BRASILEIRO DE COSTOS. 2016, Porto de Galinhas. Proceedings. Minas Gerais. 2016. p. 1-16.

GOUVÊA, A. L.; LIMA, A. F. C. Direct cost of installation, maintenance and shutdown of the patient-controlled analgesia pump. Revista da Escola de Enfermagem da Usp, [s.l.], v. 48, n. 1, p.104-109, feb. 2014. FapUNIFESP (SciELO).

GRANDO, P.; ASCARI, R. A. Victims of accidents at work treated at an urgent and emergency care center. Revista Uningà Review, Santa Catarina, V.20, n.3, pp.06-11. Oct - Dec 2014.

GROSSI, J. V. M.; CAVAZZOLA, L.T.; BREIGEIRON, R. Inguinal hernia repair: can the three main nerves of the region be identified? Journal, Jun 2015, Volume 42 N° 3 Pages 149 - 153

GURGEL JÛNIOR, G. D.; VIEIRA, M. M. Total quality and hospital administration: exploring conceptual disjunctions. Ciência e Saùde Coletiva, v.07, n.02, p. 325-334, 2002.

HERRERA, M. C.; RUIZ, L. P.; LÓPEZ, H. B. Importancia de la farmacoeconomia para la formación integral de los profesionales farmacéuticos en Cuba. Pharmacoecon Span Res Artic, Cuba, v. 11, n. 4, p.147-153, may 2014.

IZAIAS, E. M.; et al. Cost and characterization of hospital-acquired infections in the elderly. Revista Ciência & Saùde Coletiva, 19(8):3395-3402, 2014.

LIMA, L. E. A. et al. High and low frequency transcutaneous electrical nerve stimulation on the intensity of post-cesarean pain. Fisioter. Pesq., Parnaiba, v. 21, n. 3, p.243-248, jul. 2014.

LIN, J. G. et al. The effect of high and low frequency electroacupuncture in pain after lower abdominal surgery. Pain, v.99, p. 509-514, 2002.

LUIZA, V. L.; CASTRO. C. G.; NUNES, J. M. Acquisition of medicines in the public sector: the quality-cost binomial. Caderno Saùde Pùblica, v.15, n.04, p. 769-776, 1999.

MACHADO, C. L.; BRITO, R. M.; BELMONTE, L. M. Effects of the application of transcutaneous nerve electrostimulation (TENS) on pain and lung volumes in individuals undergoing cardiac surgery. Fisioterapia Reabilitaçâo, Palhoça, v. 1, n. 1, p.34-41, jun. 2017.

MACHADO, Juliana Pires; MARTINS, Ana Cristina Marques; MARTINS, Mônica Silva. Evaluating the quality of hospital care in Brazil: a systematic review. Cad. Saùde Pùblica, Rio de Janeiro, v. 29, n. 6, p. 10631082, June 2013.

MAHURE, S. A. et al. Transcutaneous electrical nerve stimulation for postoperative pain relief after arthroscopic rotator cuff repair: a prospective double-blinded randomized trial. Journal Of Shoulder And Elbow Surgery Board Of Trustees. 2017.

MARQUES, A. C. G.; et al. Characterization of accidents involving exposure to biological material in a public hospital. Rev Pesq Saùde, 15(3): 364-367, Sep-Dec, 2014.

MARTINS, C. E. A. Expenditure on medicines as a determinant of health outcomes: application of panel models to 12 European Union countries. 2015. 89f. Dissertation submitted to the Polytechnic Institute of Bragança to obtain the Master's Degree in Management of Organizations, Branch of Management of Health Units. 2015.

MARTINS, G. P.; et al. EVALUATION OF THE EFFECT OF ANESTHETIC TECHNIQUES ON ACUTE POST-OPERATIVE PAIN IN PATIENTS SUBMITTED TO INGUINAL HERNIORRAPHY. Revista Inova Saùde, Criciùma, vol. 2, n. 1, jul. 2013.

MARTINS, J. L.; CURY, E. K.; PINUS, J. Temas de cirurgia pediàtrica. Sao Paulo: Atheneu, 1997.

MARZIALE, M. H. P.; RODRIGUES, C. M. Scientific production on accidents at work involving sharps among nursing workers. Revista Latino-Americana de Enfermagem, v.10, n.04, p. 5717, 2002.

MATOS, F. V. de et al. Family and community medicine residency graduates in Minas Gerais. Revista Brasileira de Educaçâo Mèdica. v. 38, n. 2, p.198-204, jun. 2014.

MELO, J.; NASCIMENTO FILHO, V. Effects of conventional TENS on analgesic requirements in the immediate postoperative period of inguinal hernioplasty. Monograph presented to the physiotherapy course. Tiradentes University. Aracaju, 2003.

MELO, J. M. Dicionârio de especialidades farmacêuticas. Rio de Janeiro: EPUB, 2000.

MENESES, C. S.; et al. Lay action and the production of mixed public-private care maps. Ciência & Saùde Coletiva, 22(6):2013-2024, 2017.

METTEN, A. et al. The introduction of the health industrial economic complex in the development agenda: an analysis based on Kingdon's multiple flows model. Revista de Administraçâo Pùblica, [s.l.], v. 49, n. 4, p.915-936, aug. 2015.

Ministry of Health. National Hospital Care Policy (PNHOSP) within the scope of the Unified Health System (SUS), establishing guidelines for the organization of the hospital component of the Health Care Network (RAS).

MIWA, M. J.; SERAPIONI, M.; VENTURA, C. a. a. THE invisible presence of local health councils. Saùde Soc. Sâo Paulo, v.26, n.2, p.411-423, 2017.

MOREIRA, L.; TRUPPEL, Y. M.; KOZOVITS, F. G. P.; SANTOS, V. A.; ATET, V. Post-operative analgesia: an overview of pain control. Revista Dor, Jun 2013, Volume 14 N° 2 Pages 106 - 110

ODERDA, C. et al. Cost of opioid-related adverse drug events in surgical patients. Journal of Pain and Symptom Management, v.25, n.03, p. 276-83, 2003.

PADOZEVE, M. C.; FORTALEZA, C. M. Healthcare-related infections: challenges for public health in Brazil. Rev Saùde Pùblica 2014;48(6):995-1001.

PAES, A. R. M.; et al. Epidemiological study of cross infection in Intensive Care Unit. Rev Enferm UFPI. Piaui. 2014 Oct-Dec;3(4):10-7.

PAIM, R. S. P.; et al. Measurement errors and patient safety: an integrated literature review. Rev Eletrônica Gestao e Saùde. Brasilia. V. 07, n. 03, pp. 1257-70. September, 2016.

PALANCO, G. M. et al. Postoperative pain management in Spanish hospitals. A cohort study using the PAIN-OUT registry, Journal of Pain. May. 2017, doi: 10.1016/j.jpain.2017.05.006.

PALERMO, M.; ACQUAFRESCA, P. A.; BRUNO, M.; TARSITANO, F. HERNIOPLASTY WITH AND WITHOUT MESH: ANALYSIS OF

IMMEDIATE COMPLICATIONS IN A RANDOMIZED CONTROLLED CLINICAL TRIAL.ABCD. Brazilian Archives of Digestive Surgery. Sao Paulo, Sep 2015, Volume 28 N° 3 Pages 157 - 160

PEDROSO, L. M.; MELO, R. M.; SILVA JUNIOR, N. J. COMPARATIVE STUDY OF POST-OPERATIVE PAIN BETWEEN LICHTENSTEIN AND LAPAROSCOPIC SURGICAL TECHNIQUES IN THE TREATMENT OF UNILATERAL NON-RECOVERED INGUINAL HERNIA.ABCD, arq. bras. cir. dig. vol.30 no.3 Sao Paulo July/Sept. 2017.

PONKA, J. L. The hernia problem in the female. In: PONKA, J. L. Hernias on the abdominal wall. Phyladelphia: Saunders Company, 1980. p. 82-90.

Anti-crisis remedy. Revista visao saùde. Year 1 N° 01. July/Aug/Sept 2016.

ROCHA, C. R. The study of the principle of subsidiarity and the importance of local power for the development of the Unified Health System - SUS. National Seminar on social demands and public policies in contemporary society. 2016.

RUDOLPH, A. M.; KAMEI, R. K. Rudolph: principios de pediatria. Sao Paulo: Roca, 1997.

SALAZAR, R. E. M.; VILCHIS, J. E. R. Overpricing and access to medicines: the case of essential medicines in Mexico. Caderno Saùde Pùblica, v.14, n.03, p. 501-506, 1998.

SAMPAIO, L. R.; RESENDE, M. A.; PEREIRA, L. S. M. Effect of transcutaneous electrical nerve stimulation on vertebral metastatic bone pain of breast cancer patients: single case experimental study. Revista Dor, Sao Paulo, v. 17, n. 2, p.81-87, abr. 2016.

SANTOS, T. B. S.; PINTO, I. C. M. Politica Nacional de Atença Hospitalar: con(di)vergências entre normas, Conferências e estratégias do Executivo Federal. Rio de Janeiro, V. 41, N. Especial 3, P. 99-113, SET 2017.

Saùde.2017;3(3):49-58.

SCOPEL, C. T.; CHAVES, G. C. Initiatives to confront the patent barrier and the relationship with the price of medicines purchased by the Unified Health System. Cad. Saùde Pùblica 2016. 32(11):e00113815.

SILVA, C. A. L. M. An analysis of hospital spending from the point of view of supplementary healthcare. 2016. 94f. Master's dissertation - University of Brasilia. 2016.

SILVA, D. O. et al. Effects of different frequencies of transcutaneous electrical nerve stimulation on accommodation and pleasantness. Scientia Medica, Paranà, v. 24, n. 3, p.264-268, jul. 2014.

SILVA, E. N.; GALVÂO, T. F.; PEREIRA, M. G.; SILVA, M. T.. Economic evaluation studies of health technologies: a roadmap for critical analysis. Rev Panam Salud Publica. 2014;35(3):219-27

SILVA, E. N.; SILVA, M. T.; PEREIRA, M. G. Economic evaluation studies in health: definition and applicability to health systems and services. Economic Evaluation: Epidemiol. Serv. Saùde, Brasilia, v. 25, n. 1, p.205-207, jan-mar. 2016.

SILVA, K. et al. Total quality management in health services: A management model under development. Revista Eletrônica Gestâo & Saùde, Minas Gerais, v. 6, n. 1, p.617-632. 2015.

SILVA, M. B. Effectiveness of the infusion pump drug library in reducing errors in continuous venous infusion of medication. 2017. 57f.

SILVA, T. R.; MOTTA, R. F. Users' perception of health policy in primary care. Mudanças - Psicologia da Saù, 23 (2) 17-25, Jul.-Dec., 2015.

SLUKA, K. A.; WALSH, D. Transcutaneous electrical nerve stimulation: basic science mechanisms and clinical effectiveness. The Journal of Pain, v.04, n.03, p. 109-121, 2003.

SOBRINHO, F. M.; et al. Performance in the accreditation process of public hospitals in Minas Gerais/Brazil: influences on the quality of care. Rv Enfermaria Global. N. 37. Pp. 298-303. 2015.

SOUSA, M. A. S.; et al. Hospital infections related to invasive procedures in intensive care units: an integrative review. Rev. Pre. Infec. 2017.

SOUZA, N. V. D. O.; et al. Influence of neoliberalism on the organization and process of hospital nursing work. Rev Bras Enferm. 2017;70(5):912-9.

STARKS, Christopher et al. Reduction in Opioid Prescribing Using a Postoperative Pain Management Protocol Following Scrotal and Sublnguinal Surgery, Urology Practice mar. 2017.

TAYLOR, K. et all. Hernia recurrence following inguinal hernia repair in children. Journal of pediatric surgery, March 24, 2018.

TOYOTA, S.; SATAKE, T.; AMAKI, Y. Trancutaneous electrical nerve stimulation as an alternative therapy for microlaryngeal endoscopic surgery.

TRIVELATO, P. V.; et al. Evaluation of efficiency in the allocation of economic and financial resources in hospitals. Rev de adm hospitalar e inovaçâo em saùde. v. 12, n. 4 pp. 62-79. 2015.

VENTURA, M.; SILVA, N. E. K. The search for equity in access to health: the controversies of hospitalization with class difference in the SUS. Brasilia, v.4, n.1, pp. 86-102 jan/mar. 2015.

VIEIRA, F. S.; BENEVIDES, R. P. S. Os impactos do novo regime fiscal para o financiamento do sistema ùnico de saù e para a efeticaçâão do direito à saù no brasil. Institute for Applied Economic Research. N. 28. Brasilia, September 2016.

WAHLSTER, P, et al. Barriers to access and use of high cost medicines: Areview. Health Policy and Technology, 2015.

WHO, 1997a. Health reform and drug financing. Document WHO/DAP/98.3.

Geneva: WHO, 1997.

WHO, 1997b. The use of essential drugs: model list of essential drugs (Ninth list). Seven report of WHO expert Committee. Technical Report Series, n°867. Geneva: WHO, 1997.

WHO, 1998. Regional Office for Europe. The patient on focus - Special project for Newly Independent States. Program for Pharmaceuticals, 1998.

WHO, 1999. Drugs Polis - Drug Reimbursement pilot system - Special project for Newly Independent States. Drug Action Programme and Programme for Pharmaceuticals, 1999.

ZITELLI, B. J.; DAVIS, H. W. Atlas of pediatric physical diagnosis. 03. Ed. St. Louis: Mosby-Wolfe, 1997.

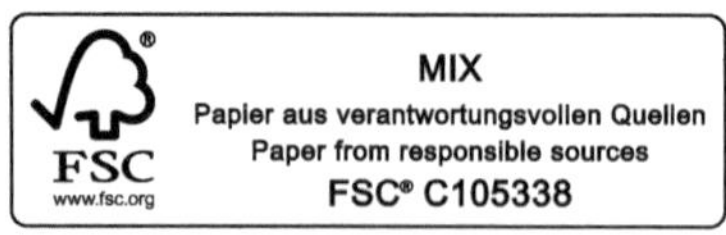

Printed by Books on Demand GmbH, Norderstedt / Germany